A Doctor's Guide to Understanding & Managing THYROID DISEASES

Dr Prabhat Das

MD, PhD, FACP

Better Health with Dr Das Series

Hardcover: 978-1-971672-40-3

Paperback ISBN**: 978-1-971672-14-4**

eBook ISBN**: 978-1-971672-15-1**

Printed in the United States of America

Disclaimer

This book is intended solely for educational and informational purposes. It is not meant to replace personal medical advice, diagnosis, or treatment.

Although I am a licensed physician, reading this book does not establish a doctor-patient relationship. Each individual's health condition, medical history, and risk factors are unique. Any medical decision should be made in partnership with your own healthcare professional who understands your specific situation.

Medical science is continually advancing. New research and updated guidelines may lead to changes in recommendations over time.

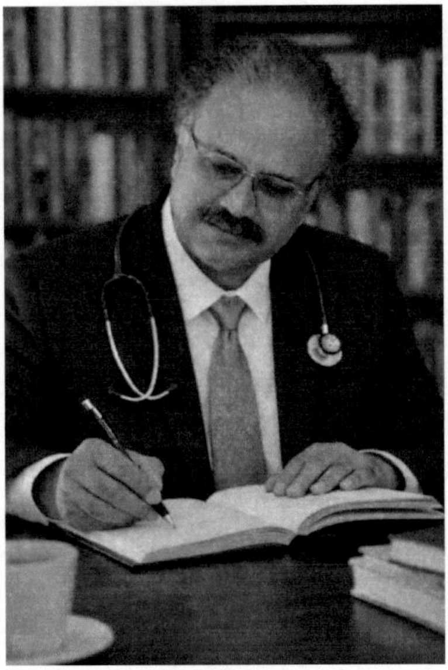

I am Dr Prabhat Das, MD, PhD, FACP. My journey in medicine began in India and, over the past thirty-five years, has continued in the United States, where I have had the privilege of caring for patients across a wide range of medical settings. I am trained in Internal Medicine, Pulmonary Diseases, and Critical Care. For me, medicine has never been just a profession. It has been a lifelong commitment shaped by learning, service, and a deep respect for the trust patients place in their physician.

Over the years, I have had the honor of caring for patients in many different situations. I have seen individuals in my office for routine concerns, treated urgent conditions in busy emergency rooms, managed serious illnesses in the hospital, and cared for critically ill patients in intensive care units. Each setting has taught me something valuable. Each patient has added to my understanding of what it truly means to care for another human being.

But one lesson has stood above all others. Medicine is not only about tests, diagnoses, or treatments. It is about people. It is about listening carefully, understanding fears that are often left unspoken, and guiding patients through uncertainty with clarity and compassion. Again and again, I have seen that what people want most is simple, trustworthy information. They want to understand what is happening in their bodies. They want to feel confident about the decisions they are making for their health and for their families.

These experiences have deeply shaped how I think about health, illness, prevention, and the human side of healing.

That is the reason behind the '**Better Health with Dr Das Series'**. Through these books, I hope to reach individuals I may never meet in person but who are searching for clear and reliable guidance. In today's world, health information is everywhere, yet much of it is confusing, overwhelming, and sometimes misleading. My goal is to cut through that noise and present important medical topics in a way that is simple, practical, and reassuring.

Every page of this series is guided by two foundations: reliable scientific knowledge and decades of real-world clinical experience. I want you, the reader, to feel informed, confident, and empowered. Not overwhelmed. Not confused. But clear about what you can do, step by step, to improve your health.

If even one reader feels less anxious, more informed, or better prepared to take control of their health after reading these books, then this work has served its purpose.

Helping people live healthier, longer, more confident and better-informed lives remains one of the greatest privileges of my life.

TABLE OF CONTENTS:

Introduction

Over the years in my medical practice, I have met many patients who walked into my office with a simple but troubling concern.

"Doctor, I just don't feel like myself."

Some were tired all the time. Some had gained weight without any clear reason. Others felt anxious, restless, or unable to sleep. A few noticed hair loss, dry skin, or a constant sense of slowing down. Many had already seen doctors, had blood tests done, and yet remained confused.

Very often, the answer was related to a small gland in the neck called the thyroid.

What makes thyroid problems challenging is not just how common they are, but how quietly they develop. The symptoms are rarely dramatic in the beginning. They creep in slowly and are easily mistaken for stress, aging, menopause, depression, or simply a busy life. Because of this, many people continue to struggle without a clear diagnosis for months, sometimes even years.

I have written this book to change that experience.

This is not a textbook. This is a conversation, the kind I have every day with my patients. My goal is to explain thyroid problems in a clear, simple, and practical way, without unnecessary medical language. I want you to understand what your thyroid does, why problems develop, how they affect your body, and most importantly, what you can do about them.

In this book, we will walk step by step through everything you need to know.

You will learn how the thyroid influences your energy, weight, mood, heart, digestion, and many other parts of your body. You will understand the difference between an underactive and an overactive thyroid. We will discuss common conditions such as Hashimoto's disease, Graves' disease, thyroid nodules, and even thyroid cancer in a calm and reassuring way.

We will also talk about something that patients often struggle with, understanding lab reports. Terms like TSH, T3, and T4 can feel confusing. I will explain them in a way that makes sense, so that when you look at your report, you feel informed rather than overwhelmed.

Just as important, we will discuss treatment in a practical way. Not just medications, but also daily habits, diet, lifestyle, and long-term care. Because in real life, managing a thyroid condition is not just about taking a pill. It is about understanding your body and working steadily with it.

One thing I want to emphasize from the very beginning is this.

Most thyroid problems can be managed very well.

With the right knowledge, proper treatment, and regular follow-up, people with thyroid conditions can live full, active, and healthy lives. I have seen this again and again in my practice.

As you read this book, I encourage you to go slowly. Think about your own symptoms and experiences. If something feels familiar, take note of it. This book is here to guide you, but your own physician will always be your best partner in making decisions about your care.

In the next chapter, we will begin with the basics. Before we talk about disease, we must first understand the normal. We will explore what the thyroid is, where it is located, and why such a small gland has such a powerful influence on your body.

Chapter 1. The Small Gland That Shapes So Much

Understanding the Thyroid and Why It Matters

When I begin discussing the thyroid with my patients, I often start with a simple observation.

Some of the most important things in the body are not always the largest or the most visible. The thyroid is a perfect example.

It is a small gland, soft, quiet, and usually unnoticed. Yet, when it begins to malfunction, the effects can be felt almost everywhere in the body.

1.1 Where the Thyroid Is and What It Looks Like

The thyroid gland sits in the front of your neck, just below the voice box. It gently wraps around the windpipe and has a shape that resembles a butterfly, with two lobes connected by a narrow bridge.

In most people, you cannot see it, and you usually cannot feel it either. It quietly does its work day after day, without drawing any attention.

But when something changes, when it enlarges, develops a lump, or starts producing too much or too little hormone, that quiet presence suddenly becomes very important.

1.2 Why Such a Small Gland Has Such a Big Role

The thyroid is part of a system in the body called the endocrine system. This system is made up of glands that produce hormones, which act like messengers.

These hormones travel through your bloodstream and tell different parts of your body how to function.

The thyroid's main job is to regulate how your body uses energy. In simple terms, it helps control the "speed" of your body.

If the thyroid is underactive, everything slows down.
If it is overactive, everything speeds up.

This is why thyroid problems can affect so many different parts of your life, from how energetic you feel to how your heart beats and how your mind works.

1.3 The Hormones Made by the Thyroid

The thyroid produces two main hormones, called T4 and T3.

T4 is produced in larger amounts and acts as a storage form. T3 is the more active hormone that your body actually uses.

Much of the T4 is converted into T3 in different tissues, depending on what your body needs at that moment.

These hormones influence many essential functions:

- How your body burns calories
- How warm or cold you feel

- How your heart functions
- How your muscles work
- How your brain processes thoughts and emotions

Even a small imbalance in these hormones can lead to noticeable changes in how you feel.

1.4 The Link Between the Thyroid and the Brain

The thyroid does not work alone. It is closely controlled by a small gland in the brain called the pituitary gland.

The pituitary produces a hormone called TSH, or thyroid-stimulating hormone. This hormone tells the thyroid how much hormone to produce.

If your thyroid hormone levels are low, the pituitary sends out more TSH to stimulate the thyroid.
If your thyroid hormone levels are high, TSH levels decrease.

This is a finely balanced system. When this balance is disturbed, thyroid problems begin to appear.

1.5 Why Thyroid Disorders Are So Common

In my practice, I have seen how frequently thyroid problems occur, especially in women and as people get older.

Some of the common reasons include:

- Autoimmune conditions, where the body mistakenly attacks the thyroid

- Family tendency or genetics
- Hormonal changes, especially around pregnancy
- Effects of certain medications
- Changes related to age

Because symptoms often develop slowly, many people do not realize early on that the thyroid may be involved.

1.6 Why This Understanding Matters to You

At first, this may seem like basic information. But in reality, it is the foundation for everything that follows.

Once you understand what the thyroid does, many confusing symptoms begin to make sense.

You begin to see connections:

- Why fatigue may not just be fatigue
- Why weight change may not be just diet
- Why mood changes may not be just stress

This understanding gives you clarity. And clarity is the first step toward taking control of your health.

Chapter Summary

- The thyroid is a small, butterfly-shaped gland located in the front of the neck.
- It produces hormones, T3 and T4, that regulate how the body uses energy.

- The pituitary gland controls the thyroid through TSH.
- The thyroid affects many body systems, including energy, heart, brain, and metabolism.
- Thyroid disorders are common and often develop gradually.

Action Plan

- Begin to familiarize yourself with basic thyroid terms such as TSH, T3, and T4.
- Pay attention to persistent changes in energy, weight, mood, or temperature tolerance.
- If you have a family history of thyroid disease, stay more alert to possible symptoms.
- Approach this topic with curiosity rather than fear. Understanding is the first step toward control.

Looking Ahead

Now that you understand what the thyroid is and why it matters, the next step is to see how it works in your everyday life.

In the next chapter, we will explore how this small gland influences your energy, weight, heart, brain, and many other functions that you experience daily.

Chapter 2. What Your Thyroid Really Does Every Day

How This Tiny Gland Affects Energy, Weight, Mood, Heart, and More

When I explain thyroid problems to patients, I often say something simple.

The thyroid does not just affect one part of your body. It influences almost everything you feel, every single day.

That is why thyroid disease can be confusing. The symptoms may appear in different ways, at different times, and in different parts of the body. Unless you see the full picture, it is easy to miss the connection.

Let us look at how the thyroid works in real life, not in theory, but in the way you experience your body every day.

2.1 The Thyroid and Your Body's Energy Use

Think of your body as a system that is constantly producing and using energy.

The thyroid helps control how fast this system runs. It regulates metabolism, which is how your body converts food into energy.

When thyroid levels are low, the system slows down.
You may feel tired, sluggish, and less active.

When thyroid levels are high, the system speeds up.
You may feel restless, overactive, and unable to relax.

This change in energy is often one of the earliest signs that something is not right.

2.2 Its Role in Weight, Temperature, and Physical Activity

Many patients come with concerns about weight. While weight depends on many factors, the thyroid plays an important role.

With an underactive thyroid:

- Weight may increase gradually
- The body feels heavier and slower

With an overactive thyroid:

- Weight may decrease
- Appetite may increase, but weight still drops

The thyroid also affects how your body handles temperature.

- Low thyroid function can make you feel unusually cold
- High thyroid function can make you feel hot and sweaty

Even your ability to tolerate daily activity changes. Things that once felt easy may start to feel tiring.

2.3 The Thyroid and the Heart

The heart responds quickly to thyroid hormones.

When thyroid function is low:

- The heart may beat more slowly
- You may feel less energetic during activity

When thyroid function is high:

- The heart may beat faster
- You may feel palpitations or a pounding sensation

In some cases, irregular heart rhythms can develop, especially if the condition is untreated.

2.4 The Thyroid and the Brain

The effect of thyroid hormones on the brain is often underestimated.

With low thyroid function, patients may experience:

- Slower thinking
- Poor concentration
- Memory problems
- Low mood or depression

With high thyroid function:

- Anxiety and irritability are common

- There is a sense of restlessness
- Sleep becomes disturbed

These changes are not just emotional. They are physical effects of hormone imbalance.

2.5 The Thyroid and Digestion, Muscles, and Skin

The thyroid also affects several everyday body functions.

- **Digestion:**
  Low thyroid function can cause constipation
  High thyroid function may cause frequent bowel movements
- **Muscles:**
  Weakness, fatigue, or cramps may occur
- **Skin and Hair:**
  Dry skin, hair thinning, or increased sweating can be early signs

These symptoms often develop slowly and may be dismissed at first.

2.6 Why Thyroid Balance Matters at Every Age

Thyroid function is important throughout life.

In younger adults:

- It affects energy, mood, and fertility

In middle age:

- It often shows up as fatigue, weight changes, or cholesterol problems

In older adults:

- Symptoms may be subtle, such as tiredness or memory changes

Because the presentation varies so much, thyroid problems can easily be overlooked.

Chapter Summary

- The thyroid affects almost every system in the body.
- It regulates metabolism, which controls energy use.
- It influences weight, temperature, heart function, brain activity, digestion, muscles, and skin.
- Low thyroid slows the body, while high thyroid speeds it up.
- Symptoms vary by age and often develop gradually.

What Does the Thyroid Control?

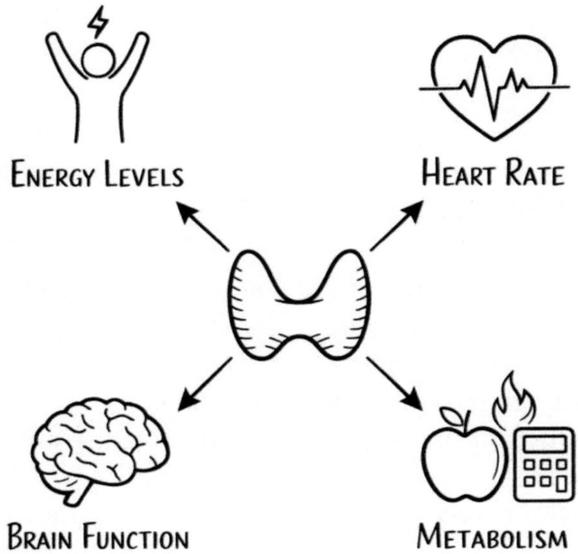

The Thyroid Affects Many Systems.

Action Plan

- Pay attention to patterns in your body, not just isolated symptoms.
- Notice ongoing fatigue, weight changes, or mood shifts.
- Be aware of changes in heart rate, temperature tolerance, and energy levels.
- Do not dismiss symptoms as just stress or aging without proper evaluation.
- Consider thyroid evaluation if multiple symptoms are present.

Looking Ahead

Now that you understand how the thyroid affects your daily life, the next question naturally arises.

Why do these problems develop in the first place?

In the next chapter, we will explore the causes of thyroid disease, who is at risk, and why these conditions are so common.

Chapter 3. When the Thyroid Starts Going Wrong

Why Thyroid Problems Develop and Who Is at Risk

After understanding how important the thyroid is in daily life, the next question most patients ask is very simple.

"Doctor, why did this happen to me?"

It is a very natural question. And the answer, in many cases, is not a single cause, but a combination of factors.

Thyroid problems usually do not appear suddenly. They develop gradually, often silently, and sometimes without any obvious reason.

3.1 The Common Causes of Thyroid Disease

There are several well-established causes of thyroid problems.

The most common is **autoimmune disease**, where the body's own immune system mistakenly targets the thyroid.

Other causes include:

- Inflammation of the thyroid (thyroiditis)
- Thyroid nodules that affect function
- Previous thyroid surgery or treatment
- Certain medications
- Iodine imbalance, though this is less common in the United States

Many patients feel they must have done something wrong. That is usually not the case. Most thyroid conditions are not caused by lifestyle mistakes.

3.2 Family History and Genetic Tendency

One pattern I often notice in practice is that thyroid disease tends to run in families.

If a parent, sibling, or close relative has thyroid problems, your risk may be higher.

This does not mean you will definitely develop the condition. But it does mean you should be more aware of early symptoms and seek evaluation when needed.

3.3 Autoimmune Thyroid Disease Explained Simply

This is one of the most important concepts to understand.

In autoimmune thyroid disease, the body's defense system becomes confused. Instead of protecting you, it begins to affect the thyroid.

Two common examples are:

- **Hashimoto's disease**, which gradually reduces thyroid function
- **Graves' disease**, which increases thyroid activity

These conditions develop over time and are not infections. They are internal immune processes.

3.4 Risk Factors You Should Know

Certain factors increase the likelihood of thyroid disease:

- Being female
- Increasing age
- Pregnancy and the period after delivery
- Presence of other autoimmune diseases
- Exposure to radiation in the neck area
- Use of certain medications

Knowing these risk factors helps in early recognition and timely treatment.

3.5 Temporary Versus Long-Term Thyroid Problems

Not all thyroid problems are permanent.

Some forms of thyroiditis may cause temporary changes in thyroid function and then improve.

Others, especially autoimmune conditions like Hashimoto's disease, often require long-term management.

Understanding this difference helps set realistic expectations.

3.6 Why Early Recognition Matters

One of the most important lessons I have learned is this.

The earlier a thyroid problem is recognized, the easier it is to manage.

Early diagnosis can:

- Reduce symptoms more quickly
- Prevent complications
- Improve overall quality of life

Delayed diagnosis, on the other hand, often leads to prolonged discomfort and unnecessary worry.

Chapter Summary

- Thyroid problems usually develop gradually and may not have a single clear cause.
- Autoimmune disease is the most common cause.
- Family history plays an important role.
- Certain risk factors increase the likelihood of thyroid disease.
- Some thyroid problems are temporary, while others require long-term care.
- Early recognition improves outcomes.

Action Plan

- Think about your family history of thyroid or autoimmune disease.

- Be aware of risk factors such as age, gender, and recent pregnancy.
- Do not ignore mild but persistent symptoms.
- Seek medical evaluation early rather than waiting for symptoms to worsen.
- Understand that thyroid disease is common and manageable.

Looking Ahead

Now that you understand why thyroid problems develop, the next step is to recognize how they show themselves.

In the next chapter, we will focus on the signs and symptoms of thyroid disease. You will learn what to watch for, what may seem subtle, and which symptoms should never be ignored.

Chapter 4. The Signs You Should Never Ignore

Common Symptoms of Thyroid Disease in Everyday Life

In my practice, I often meet patients who say something like this:

"Doctor, I knew something was not right, but I could not explain it."

That is exactly how thyroid problems often present.

They rarely start suddenly. Instead, they develop slowly, quietly, and gradually begin to affect different parts of your daily life. Because the changes are subtle at first, many people ignore them or assume they are due to stress, aging, or lifestyle.

Learning to recognize these symptoms is one of the most important steps toward getting the right diagnosis at the right time.

4.1 Symptoms That Often Develop Slowly

Thyroid problems usually do not appear overnight.

At first, the changes may be mild:

- A little more tired than usual
- Slight weight change
- Subtle mood shifts

Because these changes are gradual, you may adjust to them without realizing it. Over time, however, they begin to affect your daily routine, your work, and your overall sense of well-being.

4.2 Common Symptoms of an Underactive Thyroid

When the thyroid is underactive, the body slows down.

Patients often experience:

- Persistent fatigue and low energy
- Gradual weight gain
- Feeling cold when others feel comfortable
- Dry skin and hair thinning
- Constipation
- Slower thinking or memory problems
- Low mood or depression

These symptoms can be frustrating because they are often mistaken for lifestyle issues or emotional stress.

4.3 Common Symptoms of an Overactive Thyroid

When the thyroid is overactive, the body speeds up.

Common symptoms include:

- Unexplained weight loss
- Rapid or irregular heartbeat
- Feeling anxious, restless, or irritable
- Heat intolerance and excessive sweating

- Tremors, especially in the hands
- Difficulty sleeping
- Frequent bowel movements

These symptoms are sometimes mistaken for anxiety or heart-related conditions.

4.4 Neck Symptoms and Visible Changes

Sometimes, the thyroid itself gives visible clues.

You may notice:

- Swelling in the front of the neck
- A lump that can be felt
- A feeling of pressure in the neck
- Changes in voice, such as hoarseness
- Difficulty swallowing in more advanced cases

Any new or changing neck swelling should be evaluated by a physician.

4.5 Symptoms That Can Be Misleading

One of the biggest challenges with thyroid disease is that its symptoms overlap with many other conditions.

For example:

- Fatigue may be blamed on poor sleep
- Weight gain may be blamed on diet
- Anxiety may be attributed to stress

- Memory problems may be considered normal aging

Because of this overlap, thyroid problems are sometimes diagnosed late.

4.6 When Symptoms Need Urgent Medical Attention

While most thyroid symptoms develop slowly, some situations require prompt care.

Seek medical attention if you experience:

- Severe or persistent palpitations
- Chest pain or shortness of breath
- Sudden confusion or extreme weakness
- Rapidly increasing neck swelling
- Difficulty breathing or swallowing

These symptoms should never be ignored.

Signs & Symptoms of Thyroid Disease

- Weight Changes
- Fatigue
- Senstiivity to Cold or Heat
- Hair Loss
- Brain Fog
- Dry Skin
- Heart Palpitations
- Swelling in the Neck

Symptoms Vary Depending on the Type of Disorder

Chapter Summary

- Thyroid symptoms usually develop gradually and may be overlooked.
- An underactive thyroid slows the body, causing fatigue, weight gain, and cold intolerance.
- An overactive thyroid speeds up the body, leading to weight loss, palpitations, and anxiety.
- Neck swelling or lumps may indicate thyroid enlargement or nodules.
- Many symptoms overlap with other conditions, which can delay diagnosis.
- Some symptoms require urgent medical attention.

Action Plan

- Pay attention to persistent symptoms rather than isolated changes.
- Notice patterns such as ongoing fatigue, weight change, or mood shifts.
- Check your neck occasionally for swelling or lumps.
- Do not assume all symptoms are due to stress or aging.
- Seek medical advice if symptoms persist or worsen.
- Act promptly if severe symptoms develop.

Looking Ahead

Now that you can recognize the symptoms of thyroid disease, the next step is to understand what is happening inside your body.

In the next chapter, we will look at how thyroid problems affect different organs such as the heart, brain, muscles, skin, and digestive system. This will help you connect your symptoms with what is actually happening within your body.

Chapter 5. How Thyroid Trouble Affects the Whole Body

Its Impact on the Heart, Brain, Skin, Muscles, Digestion, Bones, and Reproductive Health

By now, you may have noticed something important.

Thyroid symptoms rarely stay confined to one part of the body. A person may feel tired, have mood changes, notice weight gain, and at the same time experience constipation or hair loss.

Patients often ask me, "Doctor, how can one small gland cause so many different problems?"

The answer is simple.

Thyroid hormones act on almost every organ in the body. When they are out of balance, the effects are widespread.

Let us look at how different parts of the body are affected.

5.1 Effects on the Heart and Circulation

The heart is very sensitive to thyroid hormones.

With an underactive thyroid:

- The heart rate may slow down
- You may feel tired with even mild activity
- Cholesterol levels may increase over time

With an overactive thyroid:

- The heart may beat faster than normal
- You may feel palpitations or a pounding sensation
- Irregular heart rhythms can develop, especially in older adults

If left untreated, these changes can put stress on the heart.

5.2 Effects on the Brain, Mood, and Sleep

The brain responds quickly to changes in thyroid hormone levels.

With low thyroid function:

- Thinking may feel slow
- Concentration becomes difficult
- Memory may be affected
- Mood may become low or depressed

With high thyroid function:

- Anxiety and irritability are common
- You may feel constantly restless
- Sleep becomes disturbed

These symptoms are often misunderstood, but they are directly related to hormone imbalance.

5.3 Effects on Muscles, Joints, and Energy Levels

Many patients describe a general sense of weakness.

With hypothyroidism:

- Muscles feel heavy and tired
- Joint stiffness and body aches are common

With hyperthyroidism:

- Muscle weakness may affect arms and legs
- Fatigue may occur despite feeling restless

This can make daily activities more difficult than usual.

5.4 Effects on Skin, Hair, and Body Temperature

Changes in skin and hair are often early signs.

With low thyroid function:

- Skin becomes dry and rough
- Hair may thin or fall more than usual
- You may feel unusually cold

With high thyroid function:

- Skin feels warm and moist
- Sweating increases
- You may feel excessively warm

These changes often develop gradually.

5.5 Effects on Digestion, Weight, and Cholesterol

The digestive system is also affected.

With hypothyroidism:

- Constipation is common
- Weight gain may occur
- Cholesterol levels may rise

With hyperthyroidism:

- Frequent bowel movements may occur
- Weight loss is common, even with normal appetite

These changes can affect overall health if not addressed.

5.6 Effects on Fertility, Pregnancy, and Hormonal Health

Thyroid health plays an important role in reproductive health.

In women:

- Menstrual cycles may become irregular
- Fertility may be affected
- Pregnancy outcomes may be impacted if thyroid levels are not controlled

In men:

- Low thyroid function may affect energy and general well-being

Proper thyroid control is especially important during pregnancy.

Chapter Summary

- Thyroid hormones affect almost every organ system.
- The heart, brain, muscles, skin, digestion, and reproductive system are all influenced.
- Symptoms often involve multiple systems at the same time.
- Understanding this helps explain why thyroid disease can feel complex.

Action Plan

- Pay attention to symptoms affecting different parts of your body.
- Do not ignore combined symptoms such as fatigue with weight or mood changes.
- If you have high cholesterol or fertility concerns, consider thyroid evaluation.
- Women planning pregnancy should ensure proper thyroid testing and control.
- Seek medical advice if multiple systems seem affected.

Looking Ahead

Now that you understand how thyroid imbalance affects the entire body, we will begin to look at specific thyroid conditions in detail.

In the next chapter, we will focus on one of the most common conditions, hypothyroidism, or an underactive thyroid. You will learn what it means, why it happens, and how it can be treated effectively.

Chapter 6. Understanding an Underactive Thyroid

A Clear Guide to Hypothyroidism

In my practice, hypothyroidism is one of the most common thyroid conditions I see.

Patients often come with a simple concern. They say, "Doctor, I feel tired all the time," or "I am gaining weight, and I don't understand why."

Sometimes they feel slow, mentally and physically. Sometimes they say, "I just don't feel like myself anymore."

Very often, the thyroid is the reason.

6.1 What Hypothyroidism Means

Hypothyroidism means that the thyroid gland is not producing enough hormone for the body's needs.

When this happens, the body slows down.

Metabolism becomes slower. Energy levels fall. Many body systems begin to function at a reduced pace.

This condition usually develops gradually, which is why it may not be recognized early.

6.2 Common Causes of Hypothyroidism

There are several causes, but a few are especially common.

- **Hashimoto's thyroiditis**
  This is the most common cause in the United States. It is an autoimmune condition where the body gradually damages the thyroid.
- **Thyroid surgery**
  Removal of part or all of the thyroid reduces hormone production.
- **Radioactive iodine treatment**
  Often used for hyperthyroidism, it can lead to reduced thyroid function later.
- **Certain medications**
  Some drugs can interfere with thyroid function.
- **Iodine imbalance**
  Less common in the United States, but still possible.

Understanding the cause helps guide long-term care.

6.3 How Hypothyroidism Feels in Daily Life

The symptoms often develop slowly and may be overlooked at first.

Common symptoms include:

- Persistent fatigue
- Weight gain
- Feeling cold
- Dry skin

- Hair thinning
- Constipation
- Slow thinking or poor concentration
- Low mood or depression

Because these symptoms are common in many conditions, diagnosis is sometimes delayed.

6.4 How It Is Diagnosed

Diagnosis is based on symptoms, examination, and blood tests.

Typically:

- TSH is elevated
- Free T4 is low or low-normal

In some cases, antibody tests are used to confirm autoimmune causes.

It is important to interpret these results along with symptoms.

6.5 What Can Happen If It Is Not Treated

Untreated hypothyroidism can lead to several problems over time:

- Increased cholesterol
- Higher risk of heart disease
- Worsening fatigue and mental slowing
- Fertility problems
- In rare cases, severe illness

The good news is that these complications are largely preventable.

6.6 The Good News About Treatment

Hypothyroidism is one of the most manageable conditions in medicine.

Treatment usually involves **levothyroxine**, which replaces the missing hormone.

With proper treatment:

- Energy improves
- Symptoms gradually resolve
- Daily life becomes normal again

Regular follow-up is important, especially in the beginning, to adjust the dose.

SYMPTOMS OF HYPOTHYROIDISM

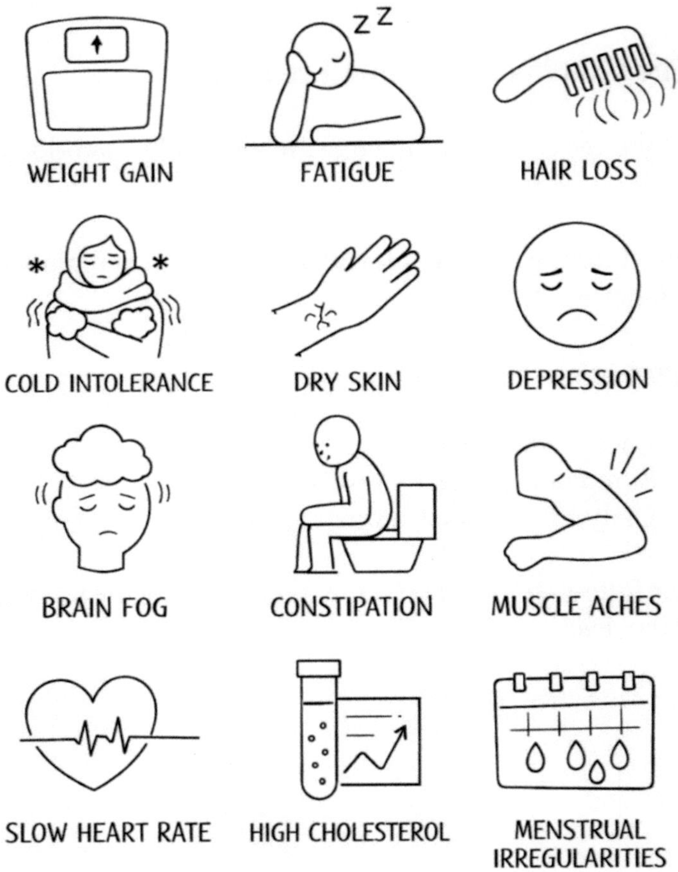

Chapter Summary

- Hypothyroidism occurs when the thyroid produces too little hormone.
- Hashimoto's disease is the most common cause.
- Symptoms include fatigue, weight gain, and slowing of body functions.
- Diagnosis is made through blood tests.
- Treatment is effective and usually straightforward.

Action Plan

- Seek evaluation if you have persistent fatigue, weight gain, or cold intolerance.
- Follow your treatment plan carefully.
- Take medication regularly and consistently.
- Be patient, improvement may take a few weeks.
- Keep regular follow-up appointments.

Looking Ahead

Now that you understand hypothyroidism, let us look at the opposite condition.

In the next chapter, we will discuss hyperthyroidism, where the thyroid becomes overactive. You will learn how it affects the body and how it can be treated effectively.

Chapter 7. Understanding an Overactive Thyroid

A Clear Guide to Hyperthyroidism

If hypothyroidism slows the body down, hyperthyroidism does the opposite.

It speeds everything up.

Patients often describe it in very simple words. They say, "Doctor, I feel like my body is running too fast," or "I feel restless all the time."

Some notice a racing heart. Others feel anxious, shaky, or unable to sleep. Many lose weight without trying.

These symptoms can feel unsettling, but once understood, this condition becomes much less frightening and much more manageable.

7.1 What Hyperthyroidism Means

Hyperthyroidism occurs when the thyroid produces more hormone than the body needs.

As a result:

- Metabolism increases

- The heart beats faster
- The nervous system becomes more active

The body enters a state where it is constantly “on,” which can be exhausting over time.

7.2 Common Causes of Hyperthyroidism

There are a few common causes.

- **Graves’ disease**
  This is the most common cause. It is an autoimmune condition where the thyroid is overstimulated.
- **Toxic nodules or multinodular goiter**
  Certain nodules produce excess hormone.
- **Thyroiditis**
  Inflammation of the thyroid can temporarily release excess hormone.
- **Excess thyroid medication**
  Taking more thyroid hormone than needed can lead to hyperthyroidism.

Each cause may require a slightly different treatment approach.

7.3 The Symptoms and Daily Struggles It Can Cause

Hyperthyroidism affects both body and mind.

Common symptoms include:

- Weight loss despite normal or increased appetite
- Rapid or irregular heartbeat

- Feeling anxious or irritable
- Heat intolerance and sweating
- Tremors, especially in the hands
- Difficulty sleeping
- Muscle weakness

Many patients feel constantly “on edge,” even when there is no obvious reason.

7.4 How Hyperthyroidism Is Diagnosed

Diagnosis is based on symptoms and blood tests.

Typically:

- TSH is low or suppressed
- T3 and/or T4 are elevated

Additional tests may include:

- Antibody tests for Graves’ disease
- Thyroid scan to identify overactive areas

These tests help determine the cause and guide treatment.

7.5 Possible Complications If Left Untreated

If hyperthyroidism is not treated, it can lead to serious problems:

- Heart rhythm problems such as atrial fibrillation
- Bone loss, increasing the risk of fractures

- Severe muscle weakness
- Rarely, a dangerous condition called thyroid storm

These complications highlight the importance of timely treatment.

7.6 Why Timely Treatment Is So Important

The good news is that hyperthyroidism can be treated effectively.

Treatment options may include:

- Medications to reduce hormone production
- Beta blockers to control symptoms
- Radioactive iodine treatment
- Surgery in selected cases

With proper treatment, symptoms improve and complications can be prevented.

SYMPTOMS OF HYPERTHYROIDISM

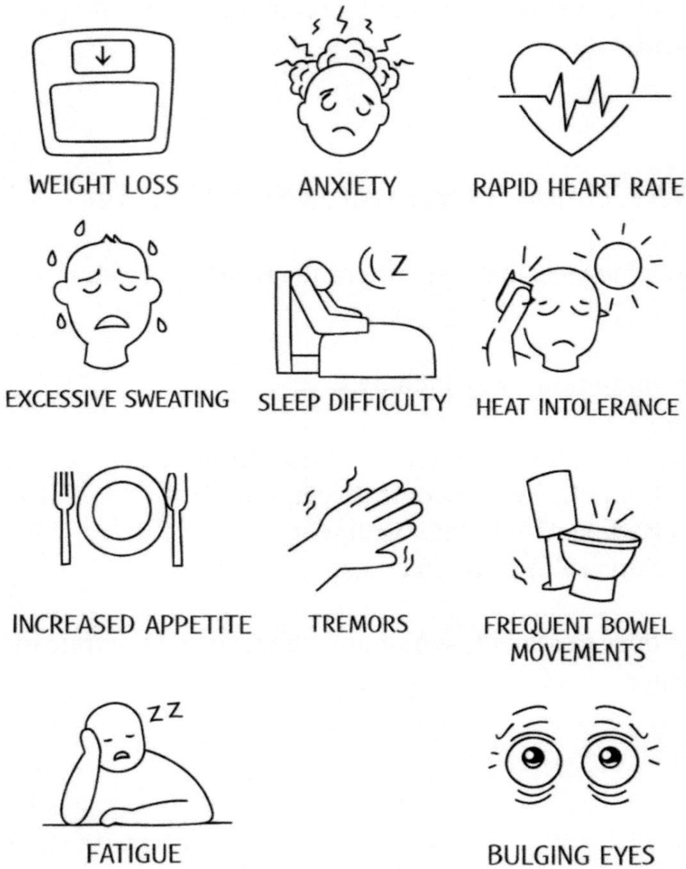

Chapter Summary

- Hyperthyroidism occurs when the thyroid produces too much hormone.
- Graves' disease is the most common cause.
- Symptoms include weight loss, palpitations, anxiety, and heat intolerance.
- Diagnosis is made through blood tests and sometimes imaging.
- Untreated hyperthyroidism can lead to serious complications.
- Effective treatments are available.

Action Plan

- Seek evaluation if you have palpitations, weight loss, or persistent anxiety.
- Do not ignore symptoms that are worsening.
- Follow your treatment plan carefully.
- Keep regular follow-up appointments.
- Seek urgent care if severe symptoms develop.

Looking Ahead

So far, we have discussed underactive and overactive thyroid conditions.

But the thyroid can be affected in other ways as well.

In the next chapter, we will explore conditions such as goiter, thyroiditis, and autoimmune thyroid diseases, helping you understand the broader picture of thyroid health.

Chapter 8. Goiter, Thyroiditis, and Autoimmune Thyroid Disease

Other Common Thyroid Disorders You Should Know

So far, we have talked about the thyroid being underactive or overactive.

But in real life, thyroid problems are not always that simple.

Many patients come with a swelling in the neck, or abnormal blood tests, and ask,
"Doctor, is this serious?"

The answer depends on understanding a few common conditions that affect the thyroid in different ways. Once you understand these, much of the confusion goes away.

8.1 What a Goiter Is

The word *goiter* simply means enlargement of the thyroid gland.

It does not tell us whether the thyroid is functioning normally, too slowly, or too fast. It only describes the size.

A goiter may:

- Be smooth and evenly enlarged

- Contain one or more nodules
- Be small and barely noticeable, or large and visible

Some people have no symptoms at all. Others may feel a fullness or pressure in the neck.

8.2 Different Causes of Goiter

There are several reasons why the thyroid may enlarge:

- Autoimmune conditions such as Hashimoto's or Graves' disease
- Multinodular goiter, where multiple nodules cause enlargement
- Hormonal stimulation over time
- Iodine imbalance, though this is uncommon in the United States

In many cases, goiter develops slowly and is discovered during a routine exam.

8.3 Thyroiditis and Inflammation of the Thyroid

Thyroiditis means inflammation of the thyroid gland.

This condition can present in different ways:

- **Silent thyroiditis**
  Mild and painless
- **Subacute thyroiditis**
  Painful thyroid with tenderness in the neck

- **Postpartum thyroiditis**
  Occurs after pregnancy
- **Drug-related thyroiditis**
  Caused by certain medications

Thyroiditis may initially cause symptoms of hyperthyroidism, followed by a phase of hypothyroidism. In many cases, it improves over time.

8.4 Hashimoto's Thyroiditis

Hashimoto's disease is one of the most common thyroid conditions.

It is an autoimmune disorder where the immune system gradually damages the thyroid gland.

Over time:

- Thyroid hormone production decreases
- Symptoms of hypothyroidism develop

This process is usually slow, and symptoms may appear gradually.

8.5 Graves' Disease

Graves' disease is the most common cause of hyperthyroidism.

In this condition:

- The immune system stimulates the thyroid to produce excess hormone
- The gland may become enlarged

Some patients also develop eye-related symptoms, which can be an important clue.

8.6 Eye Problems and Other Special Features

One unique aspect of Graves' disease is its effect on the eyes.

This condition, known as thyroid eye disease, may cause:

- Prominent or bulging eyes
- Redness and irritation
- Sensitivity to light
- Difficulty closing the eyes fully

Not all patients develop these symptoms, but when they do, they require proper medical attention.

Chapter Summary

- Goiter refers to enlargement of the thyroid and does not indicate function by itself.
- Common causes include autoimmune disease, nodules, and hormonal factors.
- Thyroiditis is inflammation of the thyroid and may be temporary or long-term.
- Hashimoto's disease leads to hypothyroidism over time.

- Graves' disease causes hyperthyroidism and may affect the eyes.
- Thyroid disorders can present in different forms and need proper evaluation.

Action Plan

- If you notice swelling or fullness in your neck, seek medical evaluation.
- Do not assume that all thyroid enlargement is dangerous, but do not ignore it.
- Be aware of symptoms such as neck pain, sudden thyroid changes, or eye problems.
- If diagnosed with an autoimmune thyroid condition, understand that long-term follow-up may be needed.
- Rely on medical advice rather than internet information for decisions.

Looking Ahead

At this point, many patients begin to worry about nodules or the possibility of cancer.

In the next chapter, we will talk about thyroid nodules, lumps, and cancer in a clear and reassuring way, helping you understand what is common, what is rare, and how to approach these findings calmly and confidently.

Chapter 9. Thyroid Nodules, Lumps, and Cancer

What They Mean and When You Should Worry

Few things create more anxiety than finding a lump in the neck.

I have seen this many times in my practice. A patient notices a swelling or is told after an ultrasound, "You have a thyroid nodule." Almost immediately, the fear of cancer comes to mind.

Let me reassure you right at the beginning.

Most thyroid nodules are **not cancerous**.

In fact, the majority are harmless and do not cause serious problems. The key is to evaluate them properly and not jump to conclusions.

9.1 What a Thyroid Nodule Is

A thyroid nodule is simply a small lump within the thyroid gland.

It can be:

- Solid

- Fluid-filled
- A mixture of both

Many nodules are discovered by chance during imaging studies done for other reasons. Others may be felt during a physical exam.

9.2 Are Most Nodules Dangerous?

This is the most important question.

The answer is reassuring.

Most thyroid nodules are benign. Only a small percentage are cancerous. Even when cancer is present, many thyroid cancers grow slowly and are highly treatable.

So the goal is not to panic, but also not to ignore.

9.3 Warning Signs That Need Proper Evaluation

Certain features deserve closer attention:

- A lump that is growing quickly
- A hard or irregular nodule
- Persistent hoarseness of voice
- Difficulty swallowing or breathing
- Enlarged lymph nodes in the neck
- History of radiation exposure

These signs do not automatically mean cancer, but they require careful evaluation.

9.4 Tests Used to Evaluate a Nodule

Evaluation is usually straightforward.

Common tests include:

- **Ultrasound**
  This is the most important imaging test. It helps assess size, shape, and structure.
- **Thyroid blood tests**
  To check overall thyroid function.
- **Fine needle aspiration (FNA) biopsy**
  A simple procedure used to collect cells from the nodule for analysis.

These tests help determine whether the nodule is benign or needs further attention.

9.5 Understanding Thyroid Cancer in Simple Terms

If cancer is diagnosed, it is natural to feel concerned.

However, it is important to understand that many thyroid cancers behave differently from other cancers.

- They often grow slowly
- They are highly treatable
- Long-term outcomes are generally very good

This is especially true when the condition is detected early and managed properly.

9.6 Living Through Evaluation Without Panic

This is one of the most important parts of this chapter.

I often tell my patients:

Do not ignore the finding.
But do not assume the worst.

Follow the evaluation step by step. Stay informed, but avoid unnecessary anxiety from unreliable sources.

Most patients go through this process smoothly and come out reassured.

THYROID CONDITIONS

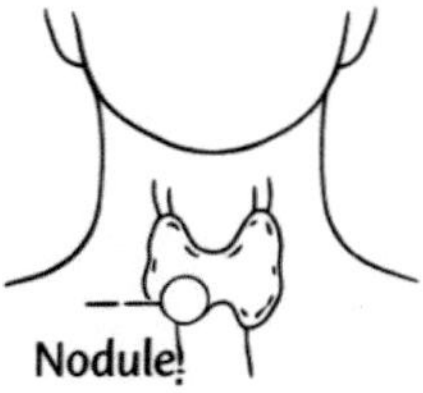

Thyroid Nodule

Lump in the thyroid gland

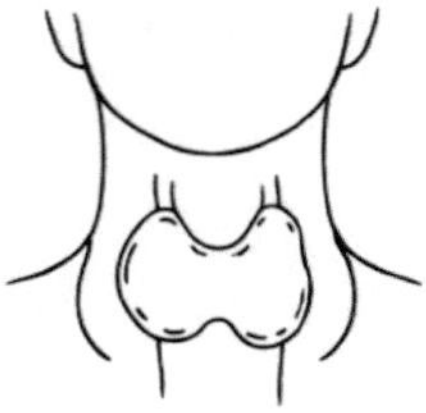

Goiter

Enlarged thyroid gland

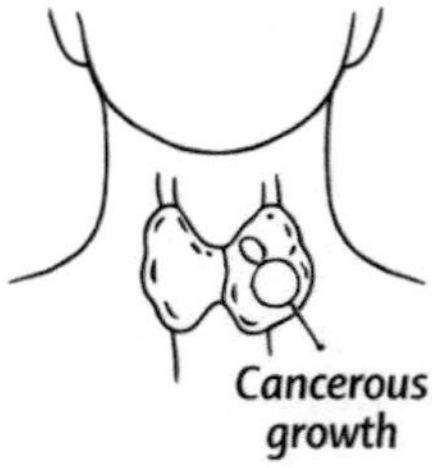

Thyroid Cancer

Malignant growth in the thyroid

SYMPTOMS

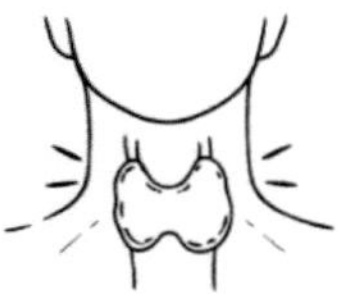

Neck Swelling

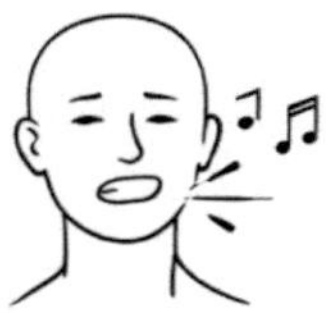

Hoarse Voice

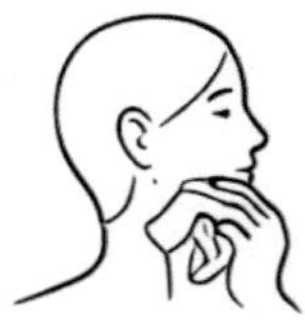

Difficulty Swallowing

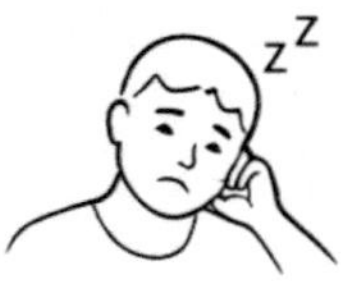

Fatigue

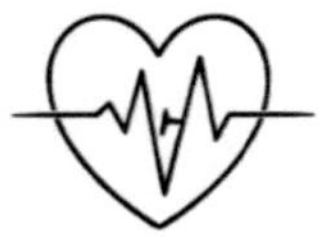

Palpitations

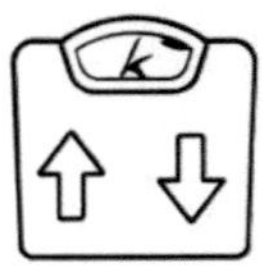

Weight Changes

Most thyroid nodules are benign. *Proper evaluation is essential.*

Chapter Summary

- Thyroid nodules are common and often discovered incidentally.
- Most nodules are benign and not dangerous.
- Certain warning signs require careful evaluation.
- Ultrasound and biopsy are key diagnostic tools.
- Many thyroid cancers are slow-growing and highly treatable.
- A calm and informed approach is essential.

Action Plan

- If you notice a lump in your neck, get it evaluated promptly.
- Do not panic, most nodules are harmless.
- Follow your doctor's recommendations for testing.
- Avoid unnecessary anxiety from unverified information.
- Keep regular follow-up if monitoring is advised.
- Stay informed and involved in your care.

Looking Ahead

Now that you understand thyroid nodules and their evaluation, the next important step is to understand how doctors put everything together to reach a diagnosis.

In the next chapter, we will walk through how thyroid problems are diagnosed, including medical history, physical examination, and different types of tests.

Chapter 10. How Doctors Diagnose Thyroid Problems

Physical Examination, Medical History, Imaging, and More

When patients come to see me with possible thyroid concerns, many expect that a single blood test will give all the answers.

In reality, diagnosis is a thoughtful process.

It begins with listening carefully, continues with a focused examination, and is supported by the right tests used in the right way. No single number tells the whole story. Good diagnosis comes from putting all the pieces together.

Let me walk you through this process, just as it happens in real clinical practice.

10.1 Why the Medical History Matters So Much

The most important step often starts with a conversation.

I ask questions such as:

- What symptoms are you experiencing?
- When did they start?
- Have they been getting worse?
- Is there a family history of thyroid disease?
- Are you taking any medications?

- Have you had any previous thyroid problems or treatments?

This information often provides the first and most important clues.

10.2 What the Physical Examination Can Show

A careful physical examination can reveal valuable signs.

During the exam, I look for:

- Enlargement of the thyroid (goiter)
- Presence of nodules or lumps
- Heart rate and rhythm
- Tremors in the hands
- Skin texture and moisture
- Reflexes and muscle strength

Sometimes, these signs strongly suggest a thyroid problem even before any test is done.

10.3 Blood Tests as the Foundation of Diagnosis

Blood tests are central to diagnosing thyroid disease.

The most important test is:

- **TSH (thyroid-stimulating hormone)**

Depending on the situation, additional tests may include:

- Free T4
- Free T3
- Thyroid antibody tests

These tests help determine whether the thyroid is underactive, overactive, or functioning normally.

10.4 Imaging Tests and When They Are Needed

Not every patient needs imaging, but it is very helpful in certain situations.

Common imaging tests include:

- **Thyroid ultrasound**
  The most commonly used imaging test. It helps evaluate size, structure, and nodules.
- **Thyroid scan**
  Used in selected cases to assess how different parts of the thyroid are functioning.

These tests provide information that blood tests alone cannot give.

10.5 Biopsy and Other Special Tests

When a thyroid nodule needs further evaluation, a biopsy may be recommended.

- **Fine needle aspiration (FNA)**
  A simple and safe procedure used to collect cells for examination.

This helps determine whether a nodule is benign or requires further treatment.

10.6 Putting the Whole Picture Together

One of the most important points to understand is this:

No single symptom or test result should be viewed alone.

Diagnosis is based on:

- Your symptoms
- Physical findings
- Blood test results
- Imaging studies

All of these are considered together to arrive at an accurate conclusion.

This is why professional evaluation is so important.

DIAGNOSIS OF THYROID PROBLEM

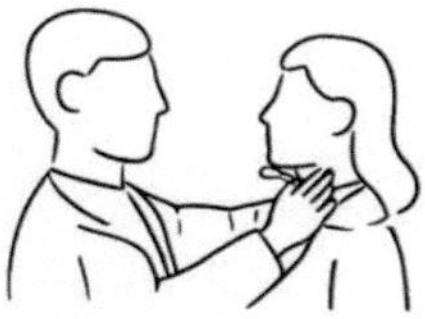

PHYSICAL EXAM

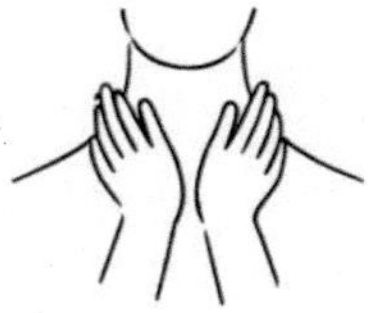

THYROID PALPATION

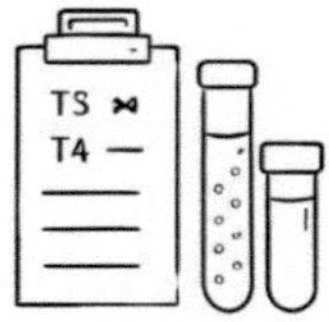

BLOOD TESTS

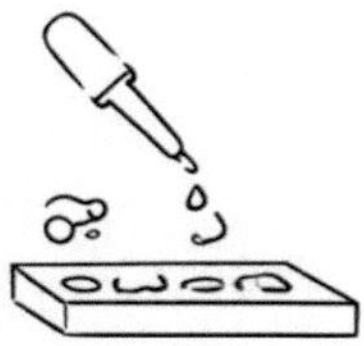

TSH TEST

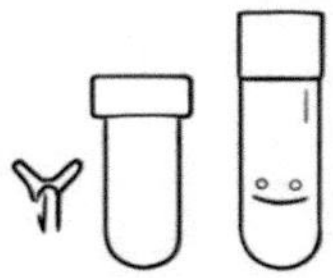

THYROID ANTIBODY TEST

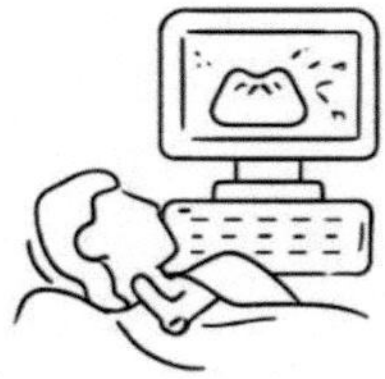

THYROID ULTRASOUND

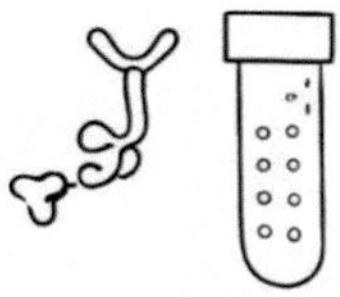

THYROID ANTIBODY TEST

RADIOACTIVE IODINE UPTAKE

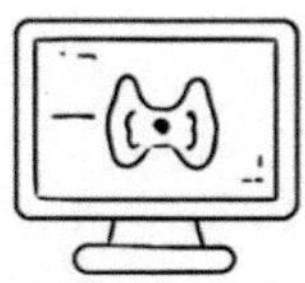

THYROID SCAN

Chapter Summary

- Diagnosis of thyroid disease involves history, examination, and tests.
- Medical history often provides the first clues.
- Physical examination can reveal important signs.
- Blood tests, especially TSH, are central to diagnosis.
- Imaging and biopsy are used when needed.
- A complete diagnosis requires combining all available information.

Action Plan

- Be prepared to describe your symptoms clearly.
- Keep a record of your reports and previous tests.
- Inform your doctor about medications and family history.
- Follow recommended investigations without delay.
- Ask questions to fully understand your diagnosis.

Looking Ahead

Now that you understand how thyroid problems are diagnosed, the next step is to understand what your test results actually mean.

In the next chapter, we will make sense of thyroid blood tests such as TSH, T3, and T4, so that you can read your reports with confidence and clarity.

Chapter 11. Making Sense of Thyroid Blood Tests

TSH, T3, T4, Antibodies, and What Your Reports Really Mean

One of the most common situations I see in my office is this.

A patient walks in with a lab report in hand and says, "Doctor, I have these results, but I don't understand what they mean."

That is completely understandable.

Thyroid reports can look confusing. There are numbers, ranges, and unfamiliar terms. But once you understand the basics, these reports become much easier to interpret.

Let us go through them step by step, in a simple and practical way.

11.1 What TSH Really Means

TSH, or thyroid-stimulating hormone, is usually the first and most important test.

It is produced by the pituitary gland in the brain and acts as a signal to the thyroid.

Think of it as a control system:

- If thyroid hormone levels are low, TSH increases to stimulate the thyroid
- If thyroid hormone levels are high, TSH decreases

So in general:

- **High TSH** suggests an underactive thyroid
- **Low TSH** suggests an overactive thyroid

This is why TSH is often the starting point in evaluation.

11.2 Understanding Free T4 and T3

While TSH gives an indirect picture, T4 and T3 tell us about actual hormone levels.

- **Free T4** is the main hormone produced by the thyroid
- **Free T3** is the more active hormone used by the body

In most situations:

- Hypothyroidism shows **low T4 with high TSH**
- Hyperthyroidism shows **high T4 or T3 with low TSH**

These tests help confirm what TSH is suggesting.

11.3 Thyroid Antibody Tests

Sometimes we need to understand the cause of the problem.

This is where antibody tests are useful.

- **Anti-TPO antibodies** are often seen in Hashimoto's disease
- **TSH receptor antibodies** are seen in Graves' disease

These tests help identify autoimmune thyroid conditions, which are very common.

11.4 Why a "Normal" Result Is Not Always the Whole Story

This is an important point.

A report marked "normal" does not always mean everything is perfect.

- Symptoms may still be present
- Values may be borderline
- Individual variation matters

This is why lab results must always be interpreted along with symptoms and clinical findings.

11.5 Common Patterns You Should Recognize

Understanding patterns makes interpretation easier:

- **Primary hypothyroidism:** High TSH, low T4
- **Subclinical hypothyroidism:** High TSH, normal T4
- **Hyperthyroidism:** Low TSH, high T4 or T3

- **Subclinical hyperthyroidism:** Low TSH, normal T4 and T3

These patterns help guide treatment decisions.

11.6 Questions You Should Ask About Your Results

To make your visit more useful, consider asking:

- What does my TSH level indicate?
- Are my T3 and T4 levels appropriate?
- Do I need treatment or monitoring?
- Should I repeat the test, and when?

Clear communication leads to better care.

BLOOD TESTS FOR THYROID & THEIR MEANING

TSH

THYROID-STIMULATING HORMONE

- High: Hypothyroidism (underactive thyroid)
- Low: Hyperthyroidism (overactive thyroid)

T4

THYROXINE

- High: Hyperthyroidism
- Low: Hypothyroidism

T3

TRIIODOTHYRONINE

- High: Hyperthyroidism
- Low: Hypothyroidism

THYROID ANTIBODIES

- High: Hashimoto's Thyroiditis (autoimmune hypothyroidism)
- High: Graves' Disease (autoimmune hyperthyroidism)

Chapter Summary

- TSH is the most important initial thyroid test.
- T3 and T4 provide direct information about hormone levels.
- Antibody tests help identify autoimmune causes.
- A “normal” result must be interpreted in context.
- Recognizing patterns helps in understanding diagnosis.

Action Plan

- Keep copies of your thyroid reports.
- Learn the basic meaning of TSH, T3, and T4.
- Do not interpret results in isolation.
- Discuss results with your physician.
- Follow recommendations for repeat testing.

Looking Ahead

Now that you understand your test results, the next step is treatment.

In the next chapter, we will discuss thyroid medications, how they work, how to take them correctly, and what to expect during treatment.

Chapter 12. Medicines for Thyroid Disease

Different Thyroid Drugs, How They Work, and What to Expect

Once a thyroid problem is diagnosed, the next question most patients ask is very direct.

“Doctor, what treatment will I need?”

And often, the concern behind that question is even more personal.

“Will I have to take medicine for life?”
“Is it safe?”

These are important questions, and they deserve clear answers.

The good news is this. Thyroid medications are among the most reliable and well-understood treatments in medicine. When used correctly, they are both safe and effective.

12.1 Thyroid Hormone Replacement for Hypothyroidism

For an underactive thyroid, the treatment is straightforward.

We replace the hormone that the body is not making in sufficient amount.

The most commonly used medication is **levothyroxine**, which is a synthetic form of T4.

Once you take it:

- Your body converts it into the active hormone T3
- Hormone levels begin to normalize
- Symptoms gradually improve

When the dose is correct, most patients feel significantly better and can return to normal daily life.

12.2 How to Take Thyroid Medicine Correctly

This is one of the most important parts of treatment.

Even a very good medication will not work properly if it is not taken correctly.

Here are the key points:

- Take the medicine **on an empty stomach**
- Take it **at the same time every day**
- Wait about **30 to 60 minutes before eating**
- Avoid taking it with calcium, iron, or certain supplements

Consistency is essential. Small changes in how you take the medicine can affect how well it works.

12.3 Medicines Used in Hyperthyroidism

For an overactive thyroid, treatment aims to reduce hormone production.

Common medications include:

- **Methimazole**
- **Propylthiouracil (PTU)**

These medicines slow down the thyroid.

In addition, **beta blockers** may be used to control symptoms such as:

- Rapid heart rate
- Tremors
- Anxiety

These do not treat the underlying cause, but they help you feel better while treatment takes effect.

12.4 Side Effects and Safety Concerns

Most thyroid medications are well tolerated.

With levothyroxine:

- Side effects are rare when the dose is correct
- Too high a dose may cause symptoms of overactive thyroid

With antithyroid medications:

- Mild side effects such as rash may occur
- Rare but serious effects include liver problems or low white blood cell count

Any unusual symptoms should be reported to your physician promptly.

12.5 Why Dose Adjustment Is Often Needed

Thyroid treatment is not always fixed.

Your body's needs may change over time due to:

- Changes in weight
- Aging
- Pregnancy
- Other medications
- Changes in thyroid function

Because of this, periodic blood tests are needed to adjust the dose and maintain balance.

12.6 Why Self-Medication Can Be Risky

In today's world, it is easy to find information online.

But not all of it is accurate.

Some patients:

- Change their dose on their own
- Start supplements without guidance

- Follow unverified advice

This can lead to under-treatment or over-treatment, both of which can be harmful.

Safe treatment requires proper medical supervision.

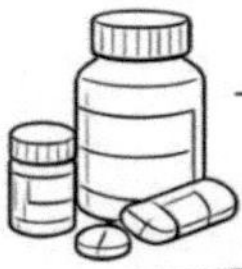

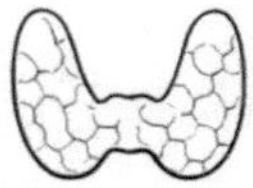

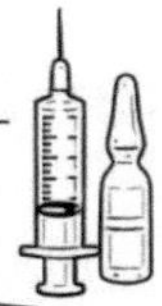

Medications for THYROID DISEASES

THYROID HORMONE REPLACEMENT

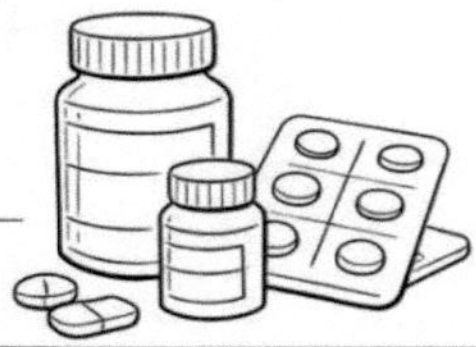

- Levothyroxine (Synthroid)
- Liothyronine (Cytomel)

Restores Low Thyroid Hormone Levels

ANTITHYROID MEDICATIONS

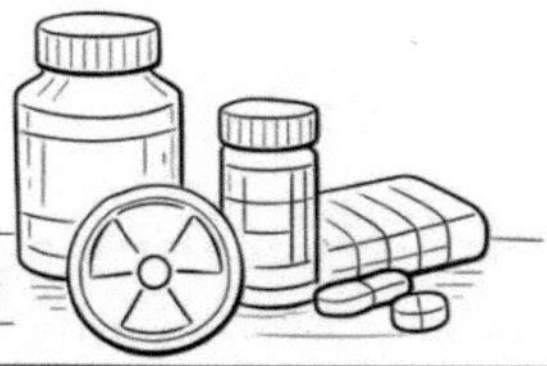

- Methimazole (Tapazole)
- Propylthiouracil (PTU)

Inhibits Excess Thyroid Hormone Production

RADIOACTIVE IODINE THERAPY

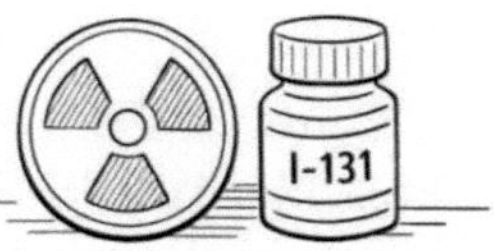

- Radioiodine (I-131)
- *Destroys Overactive Thyroid Tissue*

OTHER MEDICATIONS

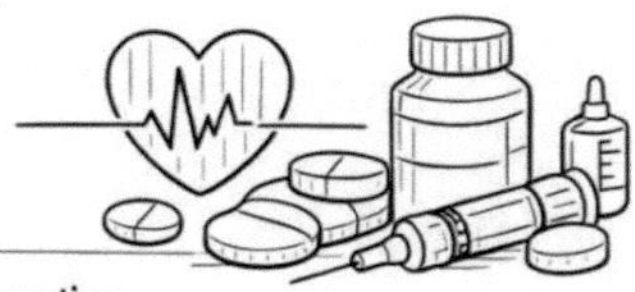

- Beta Blockers
- Steroids
- Immunosuppressants

Manage Symptoms & Inflammation

Chapter Summary

- Thyroid medications are effective and generally safe.
- Levothyroxine is the standard treatment for hypothyroidism.
- Antithyroid drugs are used in hyperthyroidism.
- Correct timing and consistency are essential.
- Dose adjustments are often needed over time.
- Self-medication can be harmful.

Action Plan

- Take your medication exactly as prescribed.
- Follow proper timing and instructions.
- Inform your doctor about other medications and supplements.
- Watch for unusual symptoms and report them early.
- Do not change your dose without medical advice.
- Keep regular follow-up appointments.

Looking Ahead

Medicines are an important part of treatment, but they are not the whole story.

In the next chapter, we will explore other important aspects of thyroid care, including diet, lifestyle, surgery, and radioactive iodine treatment.

Chapter 13. Beyond Medicines

Diet, Lifestyle, Surgery, Radioactive Iodine, and Other Treatment Options

Once patients understand their medications, the next set of questions almost always follows.

"Doctor, what should I eat?"
"Can lifestyle changes help?"
"Will I ever need surgery?"

These are very important questions.

While medicines form the foundation of thyroid treatment, they are only one part of the overall picture. Good thyroid care also includes lifestyle, nutrition, and, in some cases, additional treatments.

Let us look at these in a simple and practical way.

13.1 The Role of Food and Nutrition

Many patients hope that diet alone can correct thyroid problems.

The truth is more balanced.

Diet plays a **supportive role**, but it does not replace medical treatment in most cases.

Important points to remember:

- **Iodine** is necessary for thyroid hormone production, but both too little and too much can be harmful
- In the United States, iodine deficiency is uncommon
- A **balanced diet** with adequate protein, fruits, vegetables, and whole grains supports overall health

Extreme diets and "thyroid cure" claims should be approached with caution.

13.2 Supplements, Herbal Claims, and Internet Advice

In today's digital world, patients are often exposed to many claims about "natural thyroid treatment."

I always advise caution.

- Many supplements are not well tested
- Some may interfere with thyroid function or medications
- "Natural" does not always mean safe

Before taking any supplement, it is wise to discuss it with your physician.

13.3 Exercise, Sleep, and Stress Management

Lifestyle habits play an important supportive role.

- **Exercise** improves energy, mood, and overall health
- **Sleep** is essential, especially when thyroid imbalance affects rest
- **Stress management** helps improve well-being and reduces symptom burden

These steps do not replace treatment, but they make a meaningful difference.

13.4 When Surgery Becomes an Option

Surgery is not needed for most thyroid conditions, but it is important in certain situations:

- Large goiter causing pressure or discomfort
- Suspicious or confirmed thyroid cancer
- Hyperthyroidism not controlled with medication
- Nodules causing symptoms

Thyroid surgery is generally safe when performed by experienced surgeons.

13.5 Radioactive Iodine Treatment

Radioactive iodine (RAI) is a well-established treatment, especially for hyperthyroidism.

It works by:

- Being absorbed by thyroid cells

- Gradually reducing their activity

It is commonly used in:

- Graves' disease
- Toxic nodules

In many cases, it leads to hypothyroidism, which is then treated with hormone replacement.

13.6 A Balanced and Practical Approach

The best results come from combining:

- Proper medical treatment
- Healthy lifestyle habits
- Regular monitoring
- Good communication with your physician

There is no quick fix.

But with steady, informed care, outcomes are usually very good.

Chapter Summary

- Diet supports thyroid health but does not replace treatment.
- Supplements and "natural cures" should be approached cautiously.

- Exercise, sleep, and stress management improve well-being.
- Surgery and radioactive iodine are important options in selected cases.
- A balanced, long-term approach gives the best results.

Action Plan

- Maintain a balanced diet rather than following extreme plans.
- Avoid supplements without medical advice.
- Incorporate regular physical activity into your routine.
- Prioritize good sleep and stress control.
- Discuss all treatment options clearly with your physician.
- Focus on steady, long-term management.

Looking Ahead

Now that we have discussed treatment options beyond medication, the next step is to focus on daily life.

In the next chapter, we will talk about how to live well with a thyroid condition, including emotional health, daily routines, pregnancy, and long-term wellness.

Chapter 14. Living Well with a Thyroid Problem

Daily Habits, Emotional Health, Pregnancy, Aging, and Long-Term Wellness

After diagnosis and treatment begin, many patients ask a very honest question.

"Doctor, will I be able to live a normal life?"

My answer, in most cases, is reassuring.

Yes, you can.

With proper understanding, steady treatment, and regular follow-up, most people with thyroid disease live full, active, and satisfying lives. The key is not just medication. It is how you understand your condition and how you live with it day by day.

14.1 Adjusting Emotionally to a New Diagnosis

A diagnosis often brings mixed emotions.

Some patients feel worried. Others feel relieved to finally have an explanation. Many feel uncertain about what lies ahead.

These feelings are natural.

What helps most is:

- Understanding the condition clearly
- Knowing that it is manageable
- Building trust with your physician

As clarity improves, fear usually fades.

14.2 Daily Living with Fatigue, Mood Changes, and Body Changes

Even after treatment begins, symptoms may take time to improve.

During this period:

- Pace your daily activities
- Avoid overexertion
- Maintain a regular routine

Small steps such as light physical activity, structured daily schedules, and adequate rest can make a meaningful difference.

14.3 Special Considerations During Pregnancy

Thyroid health is especially important during pregnancy.

Proper thyroid function supports:

- The health of the mother
- The development of the baby

Women who are pregnant or planning pregnancy should:

- Have thyroid levels checked
- Follow treatment closely
- Maintain regular follow-up

Timely care helps prevent complications.

14.4 Thyroid Problems in Older Adults

In older adults, thyroid disease may present differently.

Instead of clear symptoms, there may be:

- Fatigue
- Memory changes
- Subtle changes in heart rhythm

Because symptoms are less obvious, careful evaluation and cautious treatment are important.

14.5 Work, Family Life, and Social Well-Being

Thyroid problems can affect daily routines and relationships.

You may feel:

- Less productive at work
- More emotionally sensitive
- Less socially active

Recognizing these changes helps you manage them.

Open communication with family and realistic expectations during recovery are very helpful.

14.6 Building Healthy Long-Term Habits

Living well with thyroid disease is not about quick solutions.

It is about consistency.

This includes:

- Taking medications regularly
- Keeping follow-up appointments
- Maintaining a balanced lifestyle
- Staying informed without becoming overwhelmed

Over time, these habits become part of your routine, and life begins to feel stable again.

Chapter Summary

- Most thyroid conditions are manageable with proper care.
- Emotional adjustment is an important part of the journey.
- Daily habits help manage symptoms and improve quality of life.
- Thyroid care is especially important during pregnancy and in older adults.
- Consistency is the key to long-term stability.

Action Plan

- Accept your diagnosis with understanding rather than fear.
- Build a simple, steady daily routine.
- If pregnant or planning pregnancy, ensure close monitoring.
- Communicate openly with family and adjust expectations when needed.
- Stay consistent with medication and follow-up.
- Focus on long-term balance rather than short-term perfection.

Looking Ahead

Living well with a thyroid condition depends greatly on how carefully it is monitored over time.

In the next chapter, we will discuss why regular follow-up, dose adjustment, and physician supervision are so important for maintaining long-term health and stability.

Chapter 15. Why Monitoring and Medical Supervision Matter

The Importance of Follow-Up, Dose Adjustment, and Safe Long-Term Care

One of the most important things I tell my patients is this.

Starting treatment is only the beginning.

Many patients feel better after starting medication and naturally assume that the problem is solved. But thyroid care does not end there. It is an ongoing process that requires attention, adjustment, and follow-up.

Your body is not static. It changes over time. And as it changes, your treatment may need to change as well.

15.1 Thyroid Care Is Not a One-Time Decision

Taking a thyroid medication may seem simple, but the correct dose is not always fixed.

Over time, your body's needs may change because of:

- Changes in weight
- Aging
- Pregnancy
- New medications

- Changes in your thyroid condition

What worked well before may need adjustment later.

15.2 How Often Monitoring Is Needed

Monitoring is a routine and essential part of thyroid care.

In general:

- Blood tests are checked a few weeks after starting or adjusting treatment
- Once stable, tests are done at regular intervals

The exact timing varies for each individual, but regular monitoring helps keep thyroid levels in balance.

15.3 When Dose Adjustments Are Needed

Dose changes are common and expected.

You may need adjustment if:

- Symptoms persist or return
- Weight changes significantly
- You become pregnant
- You start or stop certain medications

Even small adjustments can make a big difference in how you feel.

15.4 The Importance of Physician Supervision

In today's world, it is easy to rely on lab reports or internet information.

But thyroid care requires proper medical guidance.

A physician helps:

- Interpret test results correctly
- Identify subtle changes
- Adjust treatment safely
- Prevent complications

This partnership between you and your doctor is essential.

15.5 Avoiding Common Mistakes

Over the years, I have seen certain mistakes that can interfere with good thyroid care:

- Skipping follow-up appointments
- Stopping medication when feeling better
- Changing doses without advice
- Relying on unverified information

Avoiding these mistakes can prevent unnecessary problems.

15.6 Becoming an Informed and Confident Patient

The best outcomes happen when patients are informed and involved.

This does not mean treating yourself. It means:

- Understanding your condition
- Following medical advice
- Asking questions
- Staying consistent

A well-informed patient is more confident and safer.

Chapter Summary

- Thyroid treatment requires ongoing monitoring.
- The correct dose may change over time.
- Regular blood tests are essential.
- Physician supervision ensures safe and effective care.
- Avoiding common mistakes improves outcomes.
- Patient involvement is important for long-term success.

Action Plan

- Keep all follow-up appointments.
- Get blood tests done as recommended.
- Do not change or stop medication without advice.
- Inform your doctor about any new symptoms or medications.
- Stay informed but rely on professional guidance.
- View thyroid care as a long-term process.

Looking Ahead

We have now covered understanding, diagnosis, treatment, and daily living with thyroid disease.

In the final chapter, we will address common myths, answer frequently asked questions, and bring everything together into a clear and reassuring conclusion

Chapter 16. Myths, Questions, and the Road Ahead

Frequently Asked Questions, Common Misunderstandings, and a Hopeful Conclusion

As we come to the end of this book, I want to focus on something I have seen again and again in my practice.

Even after diagnosis and treatment, many patients still carry doubts.

They hear different opinions from friends, read conflicting advice online, and begin to wonder what is true and what is not.

This chapter is meant to clear that confusion, answer common questions, and leave you with a sense of clarity and confidence.

16.1 Common Myths About Thyroid Disease

Let us begin by addressing a few common myths.

Myth: Thyroid problems always cause weight gain
Not true. An underactive thyroid may cause weight gain, but an overactive thyroid often causes weight loss.

Myth: Thyroid disease can be cured with diet alone
Diet supports health, but most thyroid conditions require proper medical treatment.

Myth: Once you start thyroid medicine, you can never stop
This depends on the cause. Some conditions are temporary, while others require long-term treatment.

Myth: Natural supplements are safer than prescribed medicines
Not always. Some supplements may be ineffective or even harmful.

Understanding these myths helps you avoid confusion and make better decisions.

16.2 Frequently Asked Questions

Over the years, patients have asked me many similar questions.

Can I live a normal life with thyroid disease?
Yes. With proper care, most people live completely normal and active lives.

Will my symptoms go away completely?
In many cases, symptoms improve significantly, though some may take time.

Do I need lifelong treatment?
It depends on the condition. Some require long-term care, others may not.

Can thyroid problems permanently affect my weight?
Weight can be managed with treatment and lifestyle changes.

How often should I check my thyroid levels?
This varies, but regular monitoring is important.

16.3 Can Thyroid Problems Be Cured?

This is a very common question.

Some thyroid conditions are temporary and may resolve.

Others, especially autoimmune conditions, are usually long-term.

But there is an important point here.

Even if a condition is not "cured," it can be **well controlled**.

And when it is well controlled, you can live a normal and healthy life.

16.4 What Good Thyroid Care Really Looks Like

Good thyroid care is not complicated.

It includes:

- Correct diagnosis
- Appropriate treatment
- Regular follow-up
- Clear communication with your physician
- Avoiding misinformation

When these elements are in place, thyroid disease becomes manageable and predictable.

16.5 A Final Message of Reassurance

If you have been diagnosed with a thyroid condition, it is natural to feel uncertain at first.

But I want to reassure you of this.

You are not alone. This is a very common condition. It is well understood. And most importantly, it is manageable.

With the right knowledge and steady care, you can regain balance and feel like yourself again.

16.6 Conclusion: Moving Forward with Confidence

Let me leave you with a simple thought.

Thyroid disease is not something to fear.
It is something to understand.

When you understand it:

- Your symptoms make sense
- Your test results become clearer
- Your treatment feels more logical

And most importantly, you begin to take control.

Once you take control, the condition becomes a part of your life, not a limitation on it.

Chapter Summary

- Many myths about thyroid disease create confusion.
- Most thyroid conditions are manageable with proper care.
- Treatment may be temporary or long-term depending on the cause.
- Good care involves diagnosis, treatment, and regular follow-up.
- With proper management, people can live full and healthy lives.

Action Plan

- Do not rely on myths or unverified information.
- Ask questions and understand your condition clearly.
- Follow your treatment plan consistently.
- Keep regular follow-up appointments.
- Stay positive and focus on long-term health.
- Take an active role in your care.

Final Closing Message

As a physician, my goal has always been simple.

To explain clearly.
To guide honestly.
To help people feel better and live better.

Through this book, I hope I have been able to do that for you.

Take what you have learned, apply it step by step, and work closely with your physician.

You can live well.
You can stay healthy.
And you can move forward with confidence.

Appendix 1. Understanding Your Thyroid Lab Report

(Simple Guide)

When patients look at their lab reports, they often feel confused. This simple guide will help you understand the basics.

Test	What It Means	Typical Range*	If High	If Low
TSH	Signal from brain to thyroid	~0.4 – 4.0 mIU/L	Suggests underactive thyroid	Suggests overactive thyroid
Free T4	Main thyroid hormone	~0.8 – 1.8 ng/dL	May indicate overactive thyroid	May indicate underactive thyroid
Free T3	Active thyroid hormone	~2.3 – 4.2 pg/mL	Often high in hyperthyroidism	May be low in hypothyroidism
Anti-TPO Antibodies	Autoimmune activity	Negative	Suggests Hashimoto's disease	Usually not significant
TSH Receptor Antibodies	Thyroid stimulation antibodies	Negative	Suggests Graves' disease	Not relevant

*Ranges may vary slightly depending on the laboratory.

Important Points to Remember

- Do not interpret reports alone. Always discuss with your physician.
- A "normal" result does not always mean everything is perfect.
- Symptoms are just as important as numbers.
- Trends over time matter more than a single test.

Appendix 2. How to Take Thyroid Medication Correctly

Taking your medication properly is one of the most important parts of treatment. Small mistakes can affect how well the medicine works.

Daily Routine

- Take your thyroid medicine **first thing in the morning**
- Take it on an **empty stomach**
- Use a full glass of water

After Taking the Medicine

- Wait **30 to 60 minutes before eating**
- Avoid tea or coffee immediately after taking it

What to Avoid Close to Medication

Do not take these within **3 to 4 hours**:

- Calcium supplements
- Iron tablets
- Multivitamins
- Antacids

If You Miss a Dose

- Take it as soon as you remember the same day
- If it is close to the next dose, skip it
- Do not take a double dose

Important Practical Tips

- Take your medicine at the **same time every day**
- Try to stay with the **same brand** unless advised otherwise
- Inform your doctor about all other medicines and supplements
- Never change your dose on your own

Appendix 3. Your Thyroid Symptom and Health Tracker

This simple tracker can help you and your physician understand how your condition is changing over time.

You can fill this once a week.

Parameter	**Week 1**	**Week 2**	**Week 3**	**Week 4**
Energy Level (Low / Moderate / Good)				
Weight				
Mood (Low / Stable / Anxious)				
Sleep Quality (Poor / Average / Good)				
Heart Rate (Resting)				
Bowel Habits (Constipation / Normal / Frequent)				
Medication Taken Regularly (Yes/No)				

How to Use This Tracker

- Fill it once a week, not every day
- Look for patterns, not small day-to-day changes
- Bring it to your doctor visits
- Use it to explain how you are really feeling

Thank You and

Please Review the Book

Thank you for taking the time to read this book. I sincerely hope it has helped you understand your health a little more clearly and has given you practical, everyday steps you can follow with confidence. If you found this book helpful, **I would truly appreciate it if you could leave a brief and honest review.** Even a few lines sharing your experience can make a meaningful difference. Your feedback helps other readers find reliable, trustworthy health information and supports them in making better decisions for themselves and their families.

Warm regards,
Dr Prabhat Das

Continue your Healthcare Journey

Good health is a journey, not a single step. It is not achieved in one day or with one book. That is why I created the "Better Health with Dr Das" series, with each book addressing a different common condition. If you would like easy, practical guidance on other everyday health concerns, you may wish to explore the rest of books in this series.

Books in this series:

- Better Health starts Here: A Doctor's Guide to Staying Healthy After 40
- A Doctor's Easy Guide to Understanding & Managing OBESITY
- Doctor, What DIET Is Best for Me?
- Doctor, Why Can't I Lose Weight? A Doctor's Guide to safe & Sustainable Weight Loss)
- A Doctor's Easy Guide to GLP-1 for Obesity
- A Doctor's Easy Guide to Understanding & Managing HIGH BLOOD PRESSURE
- A Doctor's Guide to Living Well With DIABETES
- A Doctor's Guide to Understanding & Managing THYROID DISEASES
- A Doctor's Guide to Understanding & Managing HIGH CHOLESTEROL
- A Doctor's Practical Guide to HEART HEALTH After 40: How to Protect Your Heart & Live Longer
- A Doctor's Guide to Healing & Reversing FATTY LIVER DISEASE: Simple, Natural & Science-Based Steps to Reduce Liver Fat and Prevent Complications

- Control Your ACID REFLUX, HEARTBURN & GERD: A Doctor's Practical Guide that Works
- Live Comfortably with IRRITABLE BOWEL SYNDROME: A Doctor's Practical Guide to Understanding & Managing IBS
- A Doctor's Practical Guide to Understanding & Managing GALLBLADDER STONES & OTHER PROBLEMS
- Take Control of COPD: A Doctor's Practical Guide to Better Breathing
- Living Better Life with ASTHMA: A Doctor's Practical Guide to Asthma Control
- SLEEP APNEA & SNORING: A Doctor's Practical Guide to Better Sleep & Better Health
- KIDNEY STONES: A Doctor's Practical Guide to Prevention & Care
- Protect Your KIDNEYS: A Doctor's Practical Guide to Kidney Health & Prevention
- PROSTATE HEALTH After 40: A Doctor's Practical Guide to Early Detection & Care
- ARTHRITIS: A Doctor's Practical Guide to Pain Control & Mobility
- A Doctor's Practical Guide to Fixing BACK PAIN Step by Step
- A Doctor's Practical Guide to Understanding & Managing GOUT & URIC ACID and Preventing Complications
- HEALTHY SKIN & COMMON SKIN PROBLEMS: A Doctor's Practical Guide to Skin Care
- DEMENTIA & MEMORY LOSS: A Doctor's Practical Guide to Prevention & Management
- Doctor, Why Am I TIRED All The Time? Fixing Fatigue & Getting Your Energy Back

Printed by Libri Plureos GmbH in Hamburg,
Germany

9 781971 672403